YES, I CAN AND I WILL

INSIGHTS INTO PHYSICAL DISABILITY AND HOW TO SOLVE SOME OF ITS DAILY DILEMMAS

BY

KATHLEEN KENNEDY

THE BELLFIELD PRESS

ISBN 9780-9565548-2-6

Published by the Bellfield Press, 4 Bellfield Terrace, Edinburgh, EH15 2BJ www.gkbenterprises.org.uk
Tel. 0131 6573869

Price £3.50

Printed by McKenzie Quality Print, Kirkhill, Dyce, AB21 0GN

A CIP record for this book is available from the British library

CONTENTS

FOREWORD

Disability is a strange and ever-changing thing. Sometimes we see it as a medical issue while at other times we view it as something created by society when it acts towards disabled people with prejudice, stigma and alienating assumptions. The difficulty is perhaps that so much of what we know (or imagine we know) about the lives of those with disability tends to come from people who themselves have never had the experience of being disabled. Their attitude stems from ignorance of what disability really feel like. It is one thing to *look* at disability but quite another actually to *live* with it.

That is why this book is so important, In it, Kathleen Kennedy offers us a rich and deep insight into what it means to be described as disabled and how it may be possible to live successfully despite the many ways in which a disability makes life tricky. Being disabled does not mean that one cannot live a good and rewarding life.

Kathleen's story is sometimes tragic yet often joyful; it is always honest and enlightening. Reading her book cannot fail to change the way one looks at the world and its people. I believe this work forms an important contribution to an ongoing debate around disability issues which have crucial implications both for the church and for society in general. Kathleen has offered us a beautiful gift and a deep blessing. The question is: will we accept it?

Rev. Prof. John Swinton,
Professor in Practical Theology and Pastoral Care,
King's College,
The University of Aberdeen.

ACKNOWLEDGEMENT

I should like to acknowledge my deep gratitude to all those who helped me in the writing and publication of this book: amongst others, Professor John Swinton, who gave me continuing support and encouragement; Dr Gordon Booth, who guided me in the publishing technicalities; to Mrs Jean Baxter who readily gave up nearly every Wednesday evening to assist me with the basics of grammar; and to my godson Alasdair, who constantly gave me the inspiration to write the various chapters.

INTRODUCTION

Over the years, I have been asked numerous questions about my lifelong disability and how I have been able to overcome so many obstacles on the way to achieving a high level of personal independence. Some of these may at first sight appear insuperable barriers to others facing similar problems, but the solution frequently appears obvious once it has been discovered. The purpose of this little book therefore is to illustrate some of those difficulties and to describe the kind of solutions I have eventually found.

By reflecting on my own experiences and relating them to topics that have had recent media coverage, I hope to encourage my readers (both disabled and able-bodied) to have a broader understanding of disability in general – and not simply to view it as a series of obstacles to be overcome. This collection of short chapters is essentially an account of how I live my life from day to day.

'Yes, I can – and I will' is a phrase that I often find myself saying with great delight to those who say, 'How on earth can you possibly manage to do such things?'

Here then are some of my reflections, sometimes humorous yet always intended to provide a realistic picture of how I succeed in overcoming life's daily problems. Most of the pieces within the book can be read as short, stand-alone chapters. I was originally challenged to attempt this task by Professor John Swinton after a trip to the Scottish Parliament and subsequently by Dr Gordon Booth – both of whom know that I am always up for a challenge!

I hope and trust that what I have written may inspire others who find themselves to be in similar situations to stop feeling discouraged and to say to themselves – **'Yes, I can – and I will!'**

CLOTHING AND SHOES

I love shopping for clothes and shoes, particularly if there is a special occasion which necessitates dressing smartly, for my preference is to look well-presented at all times. Clothing and shoes are essential for everyone. This is an area of my life that has caused many an upset in the past, but I have overcome most of the difficulties by now.

All clothing and shoes that I wear and have worn in the past have had to be practicable, to allow me to put them on by myself or with very little help, as my personal independence is vital. Therein lies a major problem!

Clothing

As I have said, looking smart is imperative for me. When I look smart, I feel good and positive about myself. It has also been an important issue for me to dress like everyone else.

During my school years, this was very difficult, as the school blouses, skirts and polo shirts all had buttons. Buttons are incredibly difficult for me, particularly the small ones on school shirts. At primary school, the uniform was not so strict, provided we kept to grey or black skirts with a white blouse. I tended to wear polo shirts as I could pull these over my head, which meant there were only one or two buttons to fasten. After physical education for example, I could get away with not fastening them at all.

When I was in primary seven, I recall the fashion was for bright fluorescent leggings, which meant that, out of school, I could be dressed like all the girls of my age without any question. This was particularly memorable as we had a week away to Abernethy Outdoor Centre in the summer term. As leggings are pull-on, buttons would not be an issue. Typically, however it was a freezing, rainy week and we were all in jeans and jumpers!

Once at the academy, things were very different. Wearing the school uniform was paramount and one stood out if not dressed properly. This caused major difficulties for me, as all the blouses had buttons. Even fastening a tie was a major obstacle because of my limited dexterity, but I did have my auxiliary Alison Robbie who helped me prepare for physical education lessons. At home, my parents or my brother would always lend a hand. I used to wish there was some solution to this problem.

It is nearly twenty years since I left school, and fashions have changed so much. When I wear blouses to work or anywhere else, they are not actual blouses but v-necked tops. Sometimes they have an inset that looks like a blouse. This is now a common fashion style. Looking back on all the struggles I went through with buttons, it amazes me that today it is scarcely a problem.

Another difficulty I have with clothing may be with some zips. These are sometimes so small that they are impossible to fasten, due to my lack of hand control. When I was younger, my mum would put a key ring on some of the small zips, which helped me to grip them firmly enough to pull them up or down. As I am older now – and am not planning to set a fashion trend! – It would be slightly comical to have key rings hanging from every zip! When buying clothes I try to ensure that the zip is not in an awkward place or inaccessible for me.

Shoes

In my teenage years, it used to annoy me greatly that the girls used to wear either slip-on or high-heeled shoes and I could not, since my feet have no bridges. In order to compensate for this, I wore insoles to create a bridge. As a result, I ended up wearing plain shoes, which appeared very old-fashioned. The intention was that this would correct the positioning of my feet in the shoes, which did work for a short while. The insole did not protect the sole of the shoe for long however and I wore them out very quickly.

There was a time, in my late teenage years and into my twenties, when fashionable shoes were suitable for me. This meant I could go into a high street shop and buy a pair of shoes off the shelf. That was great but, whereas most people would buy one pair, I had to buy at least two pairs, since I would go through the soles within a week or two.

Eventually the fashion changed and once more I began to struggle to find shoes suitable for me. Yes, I could obtain them if I looked in specialist magazines or on the internet but even so I had to buy two pairs together – which was proving very expensive!

I had always wanted to find shoes with a thick sole like trainers which would alleviate the problem immensely, but I could not wear trainers to work – they would look too unsightly!

A few years ago, Mum saw a girl wearing shoes that appeared to have trainer soles, and she asked the girl what make of shoes they were. They were MBT trainers. We bought one pair to see if I would be able to walk in them, as their soles are almost round like the bottom of a ball. When we saw the price however, we did a double-take, as they are around £150 to £200 per pair! When I first tried them on, it felt as if I was balancing on a ball yet managing to stay upright. They enable one to walk quite differently from other shoes, as they help strengthen the calf muscles. The question remained, how long would it be until I went through the soles. Well, I can say that one pair of shoes has lasted me from September until the end of April and still has its soles intact, although they are beginning to look rather shabby at the front. This was such a breakthrough for me. It is unbelievable to be able to buy shoes which last so well.

Each summer, from April to September, I therefore wear MBT sandals, which I love – and my current pair still look good after three years of use.

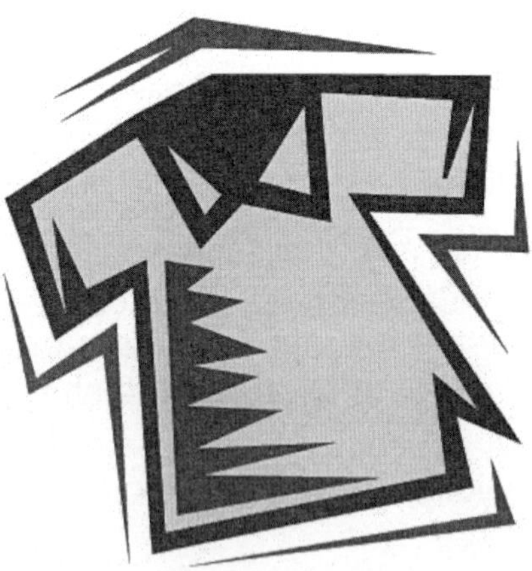

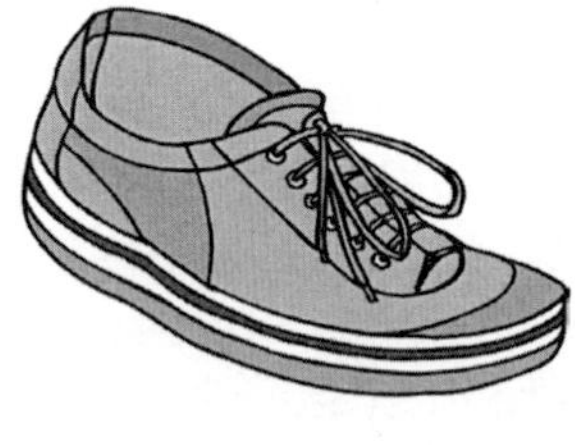

CUPS

Something as simple as the handling of cups and glasses, which most people take for granted, is one consequence of my disability, yet the problem may be disregarded by almost everyone. The fact is that attempting to hold a full cup or glass of liquid would be outwith my physical ability. My hands simply are not able to do so, due to their lack of dexterity.

Whenever I go out for a coffee (for me a cup of tea) with Mum or any of my friends, the inevitable problem of coping with cups arises. The difficulty is probably something no one assessing a business to see if it is disability-friendly would even consider.

For example, Mum and I may go into any café and order two cups of tea – nothing could be simpler, most people may think. When the tea arrives, the waitress or waiter will bring it to our table. The cups are often of the kind where I can barely get one finger around the handle and so I grip the cup with two fingers, just as I grasp a pen or pencil. Since I can barely hold the cup steady, we only fill it half full. That is fine, provided there is a teapot from which we can refill the cup, but if we are each served with only a cup of tea, we have to ask for an empty cup. This may cause consternation at first until my Mum is seen to pour half of the tea into it.

Why do businesses insist on using this type of cup? Is anyone even aware of the problems faced by the elderly, the disabled and those prone to arthritis?

Quite recently, I took the train to Edinburgh to meet the Presiding Officer at the Scottish Parliament in connection with my last book, *Living with Disability*. A friend, Professor John Swinton, was accompanying me and on the train we ordered tea and coffee. This came in throwaway cups, which are of course very flimsy. If I try to hold them, I end up squeezing so hard that I spill the tea. I was so used to this, whether at work or elsewhere, that I had brought a plastic cup with me for the journey. Nowadays we all live in a throwaway society despite all the emphasis on recycling. I appreciate that on a train it is probably easier to use disposable cups, but it seems normal procedure for most major retail coffee shops (not mentioning any names!) to use disposable cups for serving coffee, on or off the premises.

Once at Holyrood, I was sitting having a cup of tea with Professor Swinton together with my MSP Lewis Macdonald and the Presiding Officer. There I was, at the Scottish Parliament to discuss why I had written about how to cope with disability, and ironically, I had to supply my own cup. To be fair, however, I am quite sure that if my MSP had asked for a mug, one would have been found.

For me the emphasis has to be on being organised in advance, either by bringing a suitable cup with me or by having a straw for a cold drink if the glass is not suitable. Sometimes I do ask for a different cup or for a straw but until I say something people do not realise the problem.

At Home

When I was younger, I always used a Tupperware cup, which would not break if dropped, but as I grew older that wasn't very convenient. Until recently, I used a normal mug just like everyone else, but would always take only half a cup, which meant that I only had half the amount of liquid than anyone else, which caused my mouth to be permanently dry. Sometimes I would use two cups but that at times was more bother than it was worth.

At one time I had been given two tall cups, but I was somehow reluctant to use them. One day however I took them out of the cupboard and washed them. I tried one out and discovered I could hold nearly a full cup – a real breakthrough for me to find suddenly that I was able to drink a full cup without spilling. I think that the difference lies in the shape being taller rather than wider, the weight of the mug being distributed in a different way.

Glasses I could always manage, as long as they were tall and of a similar shape to the tall cups, but glass is so easily broken and the splinters go everywhere. Because I live by myself, it was not practicable for me to continue to use glass tumblers as I seemed to be dropping these constantly. I found it very hard to ensure I had swept all the glass off the floor and I was forever cutting my feet on glass after I thought I had swept up all the splinters.

So I needed to find a solution, since I wanted to continue using containers shaped like the glass tumblers but realised that this was actually becoming dangerous. Again I had to find a solution. One day I was speaking at work to my friend Heather who told me that it was possible to find plastic glasses that looked and almost felt as if they were made of real glass. I went straight out that night, bought some from the barbecue section of the supermarket, and took them home to try them out. They worked perfectly and now my glass cabinet is full of plastic glasses that look like genuine glass tumblers.

At Church

When we have communion in church, I have difficulty handling the small communion cups when they are passed round on a tray. These cups are really the size of thimbles. To take one off the tray with my lack of hand-control would imbalance the tray with the rest of the glasses. The simplest practical method for me of overcoming this is to ensure that I am sitting next to someone who is already aware of my problem. Alternatively, I might move and ask for help from someone whom I know will not make a fuss. The moment the glass is placed into my hand I have to drink from it or I will spill it. I must return the glass immediately so that I do not drop it!

What this chapter illustrates is that a problem may go unnoticed by many people yet, with some simple and sensible adjustments, everyday life can become easier for people like me through the use of a little ingenuity and experimentation.

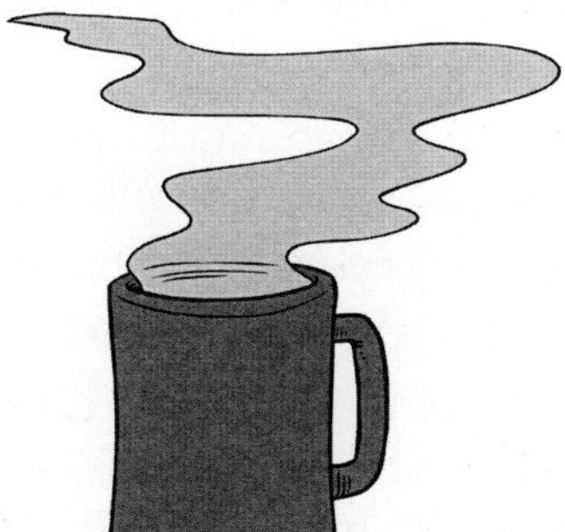

COOKING

This was a skill that I needed to learn just like everyone else, but the question was whether I would ever be able to cook safely. I imagine that this thought was always in the minds of those people who knew me as a child but, like everything else in my life, no one dared say it would be impossible – at least not in my presence. The mere suggestion would be like showing a red flag to a bull – I am so determined not to believe that anything is impossible for me!

My future independence was going to be determined by how well I could fend for myself. I could make a sandwich, but even being able to use a knife to spread butter on a roll was a major achievement – and I could hardly survive on sandwiches all the time!

I recollect baking scones and shortbread with my granny but that was not really cooking or learning to bake. It was simply following my granny's instructions. When the time came to put the baking in the oven, however, I could not risk doing so in case I burned myself. Obstacles seemed to be everywhere.

Somehow or other, I managed to work towards my Brownies' Cookery badge but I am honestly not sure how that was achieved. I must have had some help from my mother, preparing whatever was required.

Microwave ovens are, I believe, one of the greatest inventions ever made! When I was about twelve years old it seemed that everyone was buying one. Microwaves were very primitive at that time, their main purpose being for re-heating food. If my Dad arrived home late from work, his dinner was easily reheated.

When my parents ran their own grocer's shop, we quite often brought home some frozen meals, ready to put into the microwave oven. Perhaps these were not the healthiest option but at times they were by far the quickest, particularly when it might well be nine o'clock before we all sat down to eat!

However, that is not the reason I remember our first microwave: it was because I found I could heat milk in a Tupperware mug, without it becoming too hot for me to handle. I thought this was wonderful, particularly as I like hot milk on my breakfast cereal – and I also enjoy a cup of hot chocolate. This all may seem insignificant but it was certainly a major step forward for me!

At secondary school I was taught Home Economics for the first two years like everyone else, but it seemed rather pointless since my auxiliary ended up performing most of the practical work for me. However, I did learn the theory behind a well-balanced diet. That was not really the purpose of the class and back then, instead of educating people for life (as they say today) the emphasis was on all pupils complying with the standard curriculum. However, I do recall somebody querying why the school was insisting on myself (and two other pupils who were disabled) learning to cook. We all had different problems, but everyone knew that microwaves would prove to be the way forward for us.

Microwave cooking soon began to be acceptable. People spoke about "TV dinners" – yet for me this was no fad! When they first became popular, they weren't exactly healthy and any that might have been were very expensive.

On moving into my own flat, the first items to be purchased were a microwave and a fridge-freezer to store all my frozen meals. Those were vital! Dad and my brother, Calum Murdo, bought them for me, along with an ironing board which had a humorous picture of a cow on it. That makes me laugh whenever I see it!

Don't get me wrong: I do use my conventional oven, but not very often. Some foods just don't taste right when cooked in the microwave – or so I think! Unfortunately, my kitchen is small and has very little worktop space on which to lay whatever I take out of the oven. My ideal oven would be at worktop level and would have a place for hot dishes immediately next to it; but my kitchen is far too small for that.

After years of struggling to achieve a balanced diet, I now receive, once a month, a delivery organised by the local council. This consists of fourteen meals which are well-balanced, along with one or two varieties of vegetable.

This service is for the disabled and elderly, the condition being that one is able to use a microwave unaided. Yes, the meals are subsidised but the difference is unbelievable, because I feel that I have a well-balanced diet!

As you may understand from this chapter, practical obstacles are frequently overcome by advancing technology.

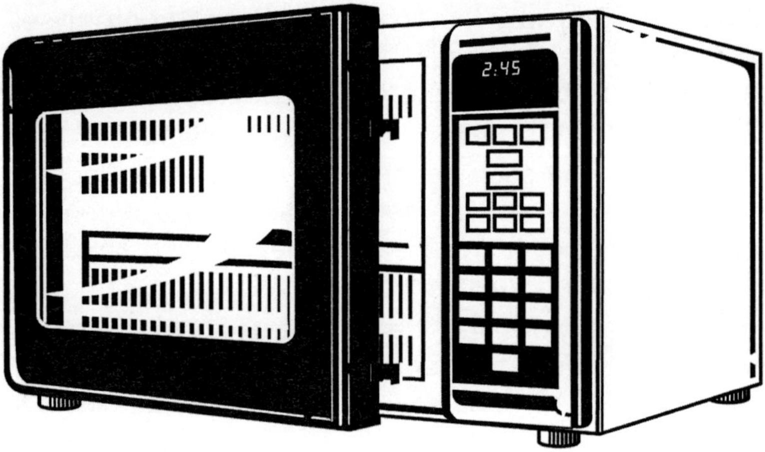

ACCESS

While pondering over writing this chapter on access, I was determined not to focus on the physical aspects of adapting a building – such as widening doors, building ramps or having disabled parking spaces in a car park. Those adaptations are extremely important and are now required by law.

However, when considering access, there is a further aspect which may well be overlooked – and that is <u>attitude</u>. The views of all those involved need to be considered. This is a vital issue but may at times be ignored.

No matter how well a building has been equipped with the suitable adaptations for disabled people, someone with a disability may still sense some unease in his or her surroundings. It may prove hard to feel accepted. Conversely, if the person with a disability is not fully accepted, because people may feel that they have 'done quite enough' by ensuring the building has been made accessible, it is difficult to break down the psychological barriers.

Once, when I was being interviewed in front of a large audience by someone who was very experienced in disability issues, I was asked about the suitability of the building in which we were sitting. In reply, I pointed out that the main difficulty was in fact getting into the building. Fortunately, this has now been rectified, but the stairs are still the only means of access to the first floor of that building.

Oh, how I dislike some church chairs, but I must say they are better than the old wooden pews! One may think churches have uncomfortable chairs intentionally to keep their parishioners awake during the sermons! Do churches realise that those with arthritis and other physical problems need comfortable seating, as they may find it difficult to sit on unsuitable chairs for long periods? Having said this, I am not suggesting that I am fat, but the simple fact is that I do need two chairs. When I am at the cinema or the theatre, this would also be the case but I cannot afford to pay for two seats! Nevertheless, in church I usually try to sit at the end of the row. This may appear unfriendly but ensures that I have enough space to move around without feeling awkward about bumping into someone sitting next to me. The more agitated I feel, the more exaggerated my movements become. I do not mind if someone is sitting on only one side of me – that is fine, but I need to ensure that I have more space on the other side. For this very reason, both my Uncle Graham and Professor Swinton were insistent that no one except for the three speakers and myself came behind the top table at my first book launch. Although they both appreciated that there was not a lot of room for all the people, due to the large number who attended, the simple fact was that I needed the extra space to avoid feeling that my movements were being restricted.

Sometimes I have found people who have become friends with me for a time seem to appreciate that certain features need to be adapted but after a short while, when the novelty wears off, they don't seem to realise that the difficulties are still there and haven't disappeared. In a way, I think it would be strange to be thought of as a novelty but, believe me, being disabled is not something that is a phase in my life: it is the largest part of my life! I have often wondered what it would be like not to be disabled just for one day. Obviously, I will never get that chance – but one can dream.

Accessibility is a more complex issue than one might think and I have intentionally covered this topic very lightly so as to show that the physical adaptations to buildings are only the start of society being truly inclusive. There is so much more to be examined to make social activities completely accessible to all.

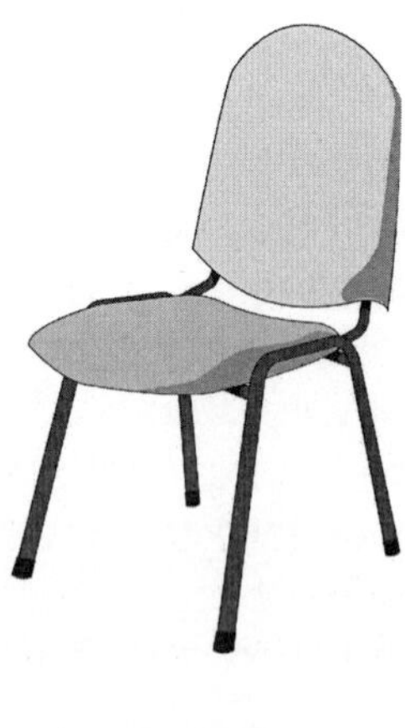

FALLING

Because of my cerebral palsy, I tend to be very unsteady on my feet compared to most adults. It often seems to me that I never grew up in physical terms. When children are learning to walk they fall a great deal – I can recollect how my own god-son was always falling when he was beginning to stand on his own feet. But of course, as they become stronger and better co-ordinated, children fall less and less frequently. For my own part, however, I have never truly grown out of the falling stage. Yes, I can indeed walk long distances, yet, because of poor balance control, my gait is always awkward and wobbly.

I often think of myself as a 'weeble' – which was a child's toy when I was young. A 'weeble' was the figure of a small man who, instead of legs, had a ball at the base. Every time one knocked the figure over, it immediately sprang up again as if it had never been knocked down. This is a good description of how resilient I am.

It is said that, as people grow into adulthood, they become more tense if they are prone to falling. With me, however, it is rather different: I may go for weeks without a fall yet suddenly fall several times in a single day. There is no point in my using a walking-stick or a 'four-wheel walker' since I don't possess the co-ordination that is needed to use such aids. I used to have a type of trolley at work to help me carry the mail until one day I fell over – and the trolley landed on top of me. Being able to fall freely when I do tumble is by far the best strategy so far as I am concerned.

It may shock friends and family to know that falling is such a frequent occurrence for me, simply because I don't mention it or admit that it is an everyday event that mostly goes unnoticed by others. How I deal with a fall depends of course on its severity. My first reaction is always to check how I feel – that is, to find out whether anything is really hurt and if so, where the damage is. If I have simply had a relatively harmless bump (as happens nine times out of ten) then I just haul myself upright and carry on as if nothing had happened. I prefer people not to draw attention to my balance difficulties and to accept them, just as I do, as an everyday event of no significance. If

I fall when in company or at work, those who are unfamiliar with the situation are often inclined to panic.

Obviously it is unusual for an adult to fall for no obvious reason; yet this is simply part of my own day-to-day living. I do, however, like the floor space to be reasonably clear of obstacles so that I don't trip unnecessarily.

I find that making a joke of myself falling is the best solution. Comments like – 'I must stop putting gin or vodka in my tea instead of milk', or 'I've just been for a trip!' – help me as well as others to make light of my falls. Humorous statements like these put my falling into context.

Whenever I have had a bad fall I like to remain where I am – even if that happens to be out of doors on the pavement – to allow time to relax and to let my body adjust to what has happened. It may take a while to figure out what (if anything) has been hurt and whether or not the damage has been serious. All too often, people around will rush to offer assistance: they mean well, of course, but don't realise that I need time and space in which to recover from my fall. Once I am ready, I will either get back on my feet unaided or else take hold of something firm to help me stand up. After a severe fall, where there may have been some actual injury, I will ask for help only after I have recovered sufficiently to tell somebody what has been hurt and to explain what kind of assistance I need.

Strangely enough, the very worst fall I ever had occurred near my mother's home in Findon one evening, as I was walking the short distance from the house to my car. Certainly it was a wild night of wind and rain but I had known that path all my life and was confident I could cope. Just as I reached the car, I fell over but quickly stood up again. I sensed that something was hurt but, ignoring my mother's pleas to come indoors, clambered painfully into the car and drove home to my flat in Aberdeen. Compared to most people, I have a high pain threshold – probably through suffering so many physical hurts over the years – and so I expected this event to be nothing out of the ordinary. Only next day, when driving to church, did I begin to realise how severe the pain in my shoulder had become. Fortunately, a friend drove me quickly to the Royal Infirmary where it was found that I had ruptured my shoulder ligament.

One of the hardest problems I have to face is when asked, 'Are you in pain?' I always tend to say, 'A bit' or, 'Just a little', in situations where someone suffering the same degree of injury might well be screaming in agony. On this occasion, once I knew I had really hurt myself, I felt quite sick and distressed. It took several months for me to recover fully and that incident really shocked those close to me, who had almost forgotten that I could actually hurt myself by falling! I remember Mum emailing my brother, Calum Murdo, to tell him that I had fallen. His response was more or less in terms of: 'So, what's new? Why are you telling me that? Doesn't she fall all the time?' Only much later, when it was fully explained to him, did he realise that I had done significant damage to myself.

As that example illustrates, I am in many ways close to being immune to physical pain, and it often needs other people to tell me before I can accept that I have a real injury. This may seem very strange but it is an important feature of my personal character, both physical and mental, and is something that I often need to explain to medical professionals as well as to friends. In addition, it may explain why I don't mention having fallen – and why those closest to me don't think anything of it either.

My advice therefore to anyone who is unsteady on their feet is to be as relaxed as possible when falling. I realise that may be easier said than done but personal experience (apart from that one bad fall) has shown that I have managed to avoid doing any real physical damage to myself! And my advice to those who may be present when a disabled person falls is to remain perfectly calm and, if it is evident that no serious harm has been done, to make light of the event and even to make a joke out of it! My granny once told me that she had fallen in town while with my aunt. The people round about kept saying, 'Get her on her feet quickly'. My aunt apparently said that that was what you did with cattle, not with a person. I think this highlights the fact that people are very different from cows and that our bodies do need time to get over the shock of falling, even when we aren't badly hurt!

SHOPPING

Shopping is a part of daily life that we all take for granted, whether it means just popping into the local shop or going to the supermarket to do a big weekly or monthly food shop. Whether we enjoy it or not, it remains an essential part of our lives. I generally enjoy shopping, even if it is only for my weekly groceries. It gives me a sense of doing something like everyone else!

Having said that, I have to admit that the experience is different for me than for the average person. I have to accept that I am likely to be stared at from the moment I go through the door, since for many people their first impression is that I am either drunk or have very little understanding of what shopping is all about. Indeed, I often feel as if I was being regarded as a potential shoplifter! That doesn't happen, however, once people in the shop actually get to know me and recognise the nature of my disability.

Sometimes on a Sunday, after having been to church, I may go and do my weekly shop and often take a friend along with me. That can prove to be a real help because, when I am alone and searching for something in particular, I may ask one of the shop assistants for help. Some may ignore me while others may scurry away as if scared. An experience of that kind may leave me feeling very frustrated indeed. I have occasionally complained and been told that I should make allowances for the reactions of the staff.

On one quite recent occasion, I happened to be in Tesco and was beginning to load my purchases on to the conveyor belt to be scanned while chatting casually to the next person in the queue, when out of nowhere (or so it seemed) the checkout girl exclaimed to me, 'How good it must be for your friend to take you out today!'

The way in which this was spoken sounded as if she thought I was being taken out of a Care Home for an hour or so and was being helped to experience how it felt to live a normal life. I proceeded to explain that I could drive my own car and held down a proper job. She looked quite stunned at that – but it left me feeling disappointed that I was not being accepted for who I am.

One of the most important issues for me, when addressing this problem, is to try to ensure that the person I am with realises how strongly I feel about being treated as a person of normal intelligence. If I am out shopping with my mother and I ask the assistant a question, they will often answer directly to Mum, who will then say, 'It isn't me who's asking or paying. It's my daughter here.'

Having a very deep faith does help me considerably to cope with situations like that. I spend considerable time reading the Bible and draw great strength from remembering the story of Moses and how God wished to use him – despite his speech impairment – to rescue a whole nation. If someone in the far distant past can be used to lead others in spite of their disability, why shouldn't I do my own shopping without the assistant assuming that I'm unable to talk sensibly to other people?

I would guess that, for both Moses and myself, the crucial factor is to have people around who simply give support and encouragement for me to carry on with the task in hand without running away or shrinking from the challenge. This is an important factor that should not be overlooked. For that reason, I avoid taking the easy way out by allowing a companion to do all the speaking or by using a home delivery service. That is no solution, particularly because I like to go shopping. Certainly I wouldn't have to struggle to take my groceries out of the car boot and carry them into the house, but being given too much assistance would deprive me of any sense of personal achievement.

In any case, expecting my companion in a shop to do all the asking would not solve the communication problem. I would lose the opportunity to help the shop assistant understand my essential normality, despite having such a profound speech defect.

Having always had a stubborn personality, I get real pleasure out of persevering and going my own way. Indeed, my determination to lead as normal a life as possible knows no bounds. In today's society, there are so many different accents and cultures that I wonder why I should feel the need to hide my speech difficulty. To rely on internet shopping would only serve to encourage the feeling that I am an embarrassment to others in public places.

Being stubborn and determined is a great help – but so also is the presence of a supportive network of friends who honestly believe my aim is not 'pie in the sky' but is a truly achievable goal. One important way in which public attitudes can be effectively tackled is of course through the education of others on the subject of disability in all its many forms. The problem is so widespread even today that it is not easy to put it right. I remember talking about this to my mother and she mentioned her own schooldays when there was one girl in her class with significant learning difficulties and who had very little speech. Mum was fascinated by the way in which that pupil could entertain herself for ages by playing in very simple ways. She was accepted for what she was – and that was fifty years ago! The point I am making is that, if society did not segregate people into different categories or give them 'labels', then there would be far greater acceptance of others, irrespective of their colour, creed, disability or mode of speaking.

But that goal may take a very long time to achieve!

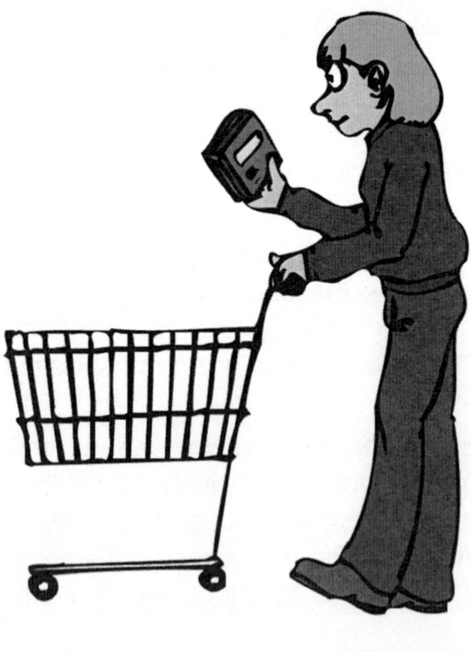

THE WORKPLACE

It is essential to regard 'work' as relating not simply to one's paid job, but also to include other activities outwith one's day-to-day employment. For my own part, work involves studying for an Open University degree, being engaged in my full-time employment, tidying up at home, organising meetings, coping with my role in the church as 'Disability Champion' (which is about raising issues concerning disability that may arise within the church) and of course my writing. Pursuing such varied activities that stimulate me both mentally or physically may eventually allow me to fulfil my real potential. At least, this is what I have gradually discovered over the years. While working in my first job, shredding paper at Stonehaven, I was also studying for my Higher National Certificate in Accounts as well as helping to count the day's takings in my parents' shop.

I greatly appreciate the fact that I do have a paid job; I regard that as a privilege because I suspect that if I applied for the post today, I would be unsuccessful – partly due to the economic climate being so difficult but also because I feel perceptions have changed and there is less readiness to employ disabled employees. This was highlighted in the House of Commons in June 2011, when one MP suggested that people who are disabled or have a mental health problem should be ready to accept less than the minimum wage. Needless to say, this view was withdrawn extremely quickly but it does indicate that the issue is a contentious one held by some influential people.

Most workplaces comply with the Disability Discrimination Act. Buildings are accessible, having lifts, ramps and disabled parking spaces. Some even give staff appropriate training on the subject of equality. Bearing in mind that every disability is unique in itself, it is hard for employers to adapt all types of work to make them available to everybody.. Of course, it is important to remember that there are many other minorities seeking employment and they all require to be treated fairly under the Equalities Act. Each minority group has its own particular needs.

Even if a company is displaying the 'two ticks' sign which implies that it is positive-thinking about disabled people, this may mean little more than that it has made the necessary basic physical adaptations to the workplace but has not considered the wider issues relating to disability.

Having achieved a HNC in Accounting and now being engaged in working towards an OU degree in Business Studies, I would love to say that I will be able to use those qualifications in my paid employment, but I often wonder whether I will have the opportunity.

I may look at a job specification and realise that I am qualified and even have the necessary experience to enable to me to apply, but there is almost always a requirement for 'good communication skills both verbal and written'. I consider my speech to be of an acceptable standard. After all, if I can talk in front of a hundred people or more, why should my oral language be an issue? Yet undoubtedly it is.

I have given much thought to the oral communication barrier. Does it also apply if someone has a pronounced local or foreign accent? As yet I have been unable to come up with a satisfactory answer to that. It is amazing that this should be an issue when we consider the range of different dialects within Britain today.

I remember once phoning a hospital to enquire about a relative, and found that I could not understand the speaker's accent – far less what was being said! Where, I wonder, do employers draw the line with regard to communication?

I have often suggested at job interviews and other meetings that if my speech is a problem for the public on the phone, there is a simple solution. It would be to prepare a recorded message to be played just before I answered the phone, explaining that I have a speech defect but will be well able to help them nevertheless. When phoning any large organisation, it is customary to hear a recorded message offering relevant information before actually being put through to someone at the other end of the line.

I often find people say how 'slow' I am, compared to others. Certainly I am physically disabled but I am not all that much slower than the average person. I enjoy a mental challenge and at my paid work there is relative little opportunity for me to be intellectually challenged – which brings us back to the point I made earlier about regarding work as broader than just one's paid employment.

If one has the right attitude, it does make a huge difference to the way in which one's paid employment is viewed. With the economy being so difficult just now, employers may pick and choose whom they are willing to employ and naturally they will pick the most suitable person for the job, whether disabled or not!

Another factor to consider when I am applying for a job is whether I will be given adequate support. For instance, I have three friends who work in the same building as I do and who always support me emotionally. Marion, with whom I have had my tea break for the past seventeen years, is someone in whom I can always confide if I am worried – which is a natural thing to do at coffee break. Another friend, Heather, also has coffee with Marion and myself, but Heather's friendship is of a different kind, because we grew up in the same area and we have many acquaintances in common. Heather, however, does something for me that I truly appreciate: every morning, just after she comes in, she goes and brings me a cup of tea. That makes such a difference to my mornings! There is one other close friend at work, Alan Campbell, who is always there to give me good advice, whether it be work-related or a church matter. As you see, it is important to have friends in the workplace who share my vision of leading a 'normal' working life, albeit with a degree of emotional support.

As I mentioned earlier, I am a 'Disability Champion' within my church, which means that I am responsible for raising any issues pertaining to disability that may arise and suggesting how they may be overcome. In this role, I report directly to Professor Swinton, who will then bring these matters to the attention of the eldership or the congregation. This happens in different ways – sometimes through participating with Professor Swinton during a service or perhaps by producing informative material for leaflets or posters. This role also involves being part of a wider church group, known as the *Welcome Church Forum*. This is designed to help faith communities in supporting families throughout Aberdeen who have children with learning disabilities. The demands placed upon the 'Disability Champion' can prove extremely diverse, depending on the specific needs of the family concerned. An awareness of this role would be potentially beneficial to many employers, through designating an employee as the specific point of contact for anyone seeking advice.

The kind of work in which I would like eventually to be involved would encourage employers to think positively and to be proactive in employing disabled people – not employing them simply to carry out menial tasks but enabling them to contribute constructively to the work environment. This would entail liaising with many different groups, but it would also require working on my own initiative, something which would suit me very well.

As I have said, I greatly enjoy being mentally challenged, and whether this occurs through studying, performing disability work at church or even writing, it all helps me to feel positive about myself and allows others to see how much I am capable of doing.

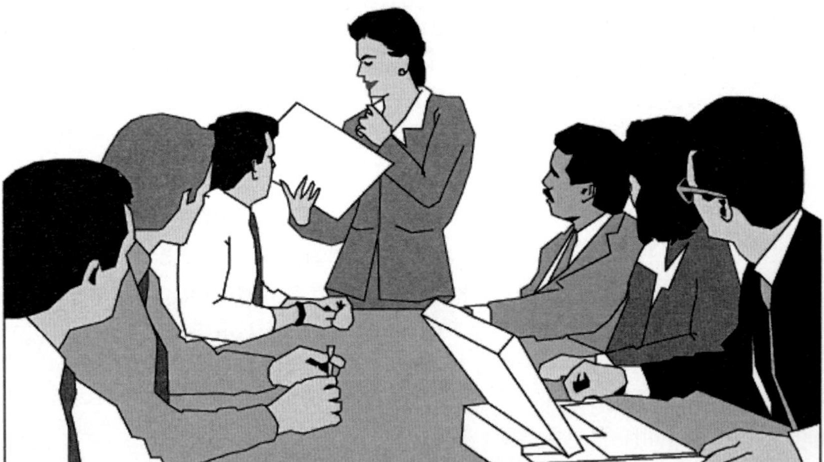

COMPUTERS

On thinking back to thirty years ago, I recall that my first electric typewriter took up almost the whole of the space on our dining-room table. Nowadays small keyboards are fashionable. What a huge difference!

I was about three years old when given my first typewriter, the reason being that it was never envisaged I would be able to write, due to my lack of dexterity. My difficulty with hand control has always been so evident that, when I received that first typewriter, a metal grid was placed over the keys to define the location for my fingers. I wonder what would happen today? Who would have thought that now I am able to text on the small keypad of my mobile phone?

I used to imagine a typewriter which would enable me to delete words and letters that I had typed at the top of the paper, even when I was working at the bottom of the page. As a child, I could see my own mistakes but nothing really could have helped me to correct them. Tippex was not an option for me. I then started to write by hand, since typewriters just seemed to be more labour than they were worth!

As computers became more readily available, my parents bought one for the family. The computer was the Sharp MZ700 and naturally it was purchased from my Uncle Graham's shop. Yes, we all played games on it but what frustrated me was that I could now type on to a television screen and correct what I had typed, yet we had no printer attached to the computer. Besides, the software still was not sufficiently sophisticated to allow this.

My perception of a typewriter in those days matches my concept of the computer now – simply as a writing tool. I have no interest in how it works as long as I can produce my written work more quickly than by writing. If this wasn't the case, why bother with them?

Not long after my parents had purchased the home computer, my educational psychologist, Gordon Booth, arranged for me to have a portable computer. This had a small screen incorporated in the keyboard. Ten characters could be displayed on it before printing it out on paper – a real breakthrough, but still not as fast as writing! I persevered on and off for some years, but it was not ideal and carrying it back and forth from home to school was another obstacle to be overcome. It still seemed to be giving me more work than actually assisting with my writing.

Just around the time that I moved into third year at secondary school, my parents bought a word processor which was compatible with the one at school. This made such a difference. Now I could carry a disc with my work on it and use it both at home and in school. Being able to type my essays made life easier than having them scribed for me or attempting to handwrite them. In exams, I still had a scribe (apart from my Accounts exams), as my uncle had adapted a spreadsheet to meet with the criteria for those exams – which stipulated that no calculations were to be done for me!

By the end of my school days, computers were very much part of my life, but some people knew I had no real interest in them apart from providing me with the mechanics of a writing tool. This is actually an important issue to emphasise as people often assume that I want to work solely with computers. Technology exists to help us but it is not a substitute for personal intelligence.

When I began work, not everyone possessed a computer. Most of my work however was done on the computer. This tended to be data-inputting, which was adequate for an eighteen year old. Gradually I became involved in other administrative duties but the common perception people still have about me is that I can only input data. Should anyone think this of someone who has an HNC or is studying for an honours degree with the Open University?

I do agree that computers have had a major impact on my life, but I believe most people today would say this. Yet these machines are only as clever as the persons using them!

Today, when studying at home, I have my laptop connected to a keyboard which is easier to type on and to correct, since the keyboard has larger keys than the laptop. This would be unremarkable, except for one item that I describe under Communication – and this is the software which reads back to me what I have typed. My laptop is not adapted in any other way.

As you will understand from what I have argued above, computers may certainly help someone like me who is faced with many physical challenges, but it is important that disabled people are not stereotyped. Do not imagine that they cannot achieve anything unless they are sitting in front of the computer screen!

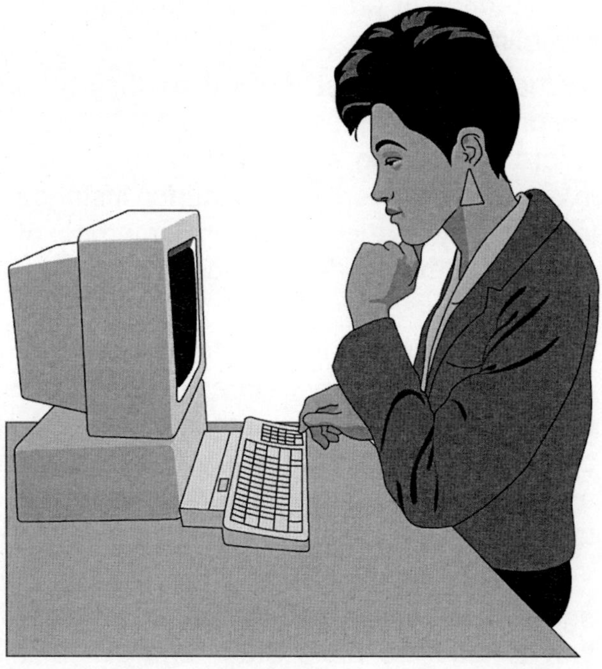

APPEARANCE

When I was young and growing up, there was always a great emphasis upon girls looking like models. The stereotype of a model then was of a young woman who was tall, slim and very glamorous. Every girl seemed to aim to be just like that. I knew from a very early age that this was an impossible goal for me. I was already beginning to be judged as someone who *looked* different. In my Open University study, I recently finished a short module on psychology and one of the sections there dealt with how first impressions encourage people to categorise others.

Try to imagine what it is like to meet someone who has difficulty walking straight and who often sits awkwardly and has a major speech defect. The first thing which may come into your mind is that this person is either drunk or has some major learning difficulty and who therefore does not realise how awkward their movements appear. This means for me that I am already being judged and put into a conceptual "box " into which I do not really fit. Overcoming this hurdle can prove a major problem: sometimes I succeed and sometimes I fail.

When people meet me, I think they are often embarrassed and are unsure how to react, particularly if it occurs in an informal setting where there is no set format or structure. When people meet me in an Open University tutorial, for instance, I find they accept me immediately, as they know I am a member of the course and so must possess some academic understanding. Like them, I fully intend to pass the course!

This has helped build my confidence. When I meet people socially or even at work, they frequently do not seem able to see past my disability. The only way around this is if someone is there who already knows me and who will show the others the way in which I am to able to communicate orally, if they would only be prepared to take some time to listen to what I am saying.

I recall being in a small Church Bible Study group some years ago, where we were studying the Book of Hebrews. It came to my turn to lead the Bible Study and one of the women kept asking me whether I would manage! I naturally said 'yes'. When the time came, I found I had prepared a more in-depth Bible Study than we normally had, so requiring two evenings instead of one. The woman who had asked me whether I would manage could not believe I had the mental capacity to do that. She had judged me according to my outward appearance, not on what I had been saying when I had been participating on a weekly basis.

I fully understand why people judge me on the basis of my appearance and therefore assume I am not able to understand many things. Unbeknown to my family, I have struggled with my appearance for over thirty years. It was not until I heard a sermon relating to the fact that the Bible states that God sees His whole creation as beautiful – and that includes us humans – that I realised how my faith could help me accept my appearance. I must admit I am only now beginning to feel positive about myself. That sermon was preached in February 2008, but it is a long process. I had a very negative image of myself when growing into adulthood, and I was often abused verbally for my appearance. Only when we really begin to see what beauty there is in each other and learn to start to appreciate the differences, will things improve.

PHOTOGRAPHS

When I look back at my old school photos or any other photographs where I have been told to smile, I feel the picture over-emphasises my disability. If asked to smile, I cannot do so on request because of my cerebral palsy. This can lead to great disappointment when people are taking photos, since I either look very stern or else seem not to be in full control of my facial movements. When I was having my picture taken for my last book, someone suggested that I should have a professional portrait. In the past, when I have had a photograph taken by an expert, it may actually turn out worse because they always ask me to smile – which accentuates the disability. I find that when I have my photo taken along with my brother Calum Murdo or my god-son Alisdair, the results turn out very well – perhaps because, when I am with either of them, I am smiling quite naturally. At my first book launch, I recall having my picture taken along with the Lord Provost, and the cameraman asking me to look at him, while my Uncle Graham was shouting for me to look directly at Professor Swinton who was standing next to the photographer and smiling at me. This is a technique which my family have learnt over many years: it is better for me not to face the camera, but to smile naturally at someone or something beside it. Thankfully, Professor Swinton had already been aware that this was a difficulty that some disabled people have. Without having to explain, he was already in position! Believe me, you can tell the significant difference between those photos and the ones taken at Holyrood: these were more formal and it wasn't appropriate for Professor Swinton to stand next to the camera for the photo being taken with the Presiding Officer – nor the second photo with my MSP, Lewis Macdonald, the Presiding Officer and Professor Swinton. It is a simple technique which makes such a huge difference whenever I am having my photo taken.

LAUGHING

I love to laugh but, when I do so, it is not always at the appropriate moment, since I may laugh when nervous or even when scared. I have heard it said that no one laughs quite as much as I do, as sometimes when I begin to laugh, I simply can't stop. Quite honestly, I just go on and on!

In primary school, my nickname was 'giggle-pot' – as I could not stop laughing, yet laughing can sometimes put me into dangerous situations – I may lose my sense of balance if standing upright. There are so many occasions when I have begun to laugh and have ended up in a heap on the floor, which is just hilarious for other people – and myself: but the downside of this is that, once I have stopped laughing, I may find that I have hurt myself without realising it.

My brother, Calum Murdo, merely has to raise one finger to indicate that he intends to tickle me and I find I'm unable to retain my composure. I burst out laughing and fall over. This is great fun, but it demonstrates how much my emotions affect my balance and even my spatial awareness.

As I have said, I love to laugh and this may sometimes confuse people. At times I giggle quite inappropriately – I consider it funny for example, when someone in church reads out an important notice in very formal and solemn language. I find that it is still more hilarious when the speaker is someone I know well.

In the summer of 2011, a situation was reported in the press concerning a boy with autism. His parents were asked to remove him from a theatre in London as he was making undue noise. Certainly, this was being highlighted in the media and well publicised, with the theatre offering an apology, but that could well have been me! I can't avoid laughing occasionally at the wrong time and, since my voice is always louder than others, whispering is out of the question for me!

As this brief analysis illustrates, a sense of humour is always essential when one has a disability.

SPEAKING

Throughout my life, I have had to deal with various specialists in speech and language, so am very aware of how people talk formally about my language and other issues surrounding my well-being in the context of the spoken word. This has inevitably placed a greater emphasis on how I find it easier to talk formally rather than casually.

If I had the choice, I would prefer in fact to talk using formal language. That was always the way in which my parents, brother and uncle addressed me whenever they discussed important world issues such as current affairs. I find that kind of language relatively easy to use as it has a logical structure and leads to a focal point. I was always expected to take part in those family conversations at an age-appropriate level. This perhaps was because, as a family, we were all practical and business-minded. When I was younger, both my parents and my uncle kept shops, so small-talk was only for the customers. Unfortunately, my lack of ability in this area has proved to be a major drawback when I am attempting to socialise with people at work, in church or elsewhere. When someone is chatting about what they are cooking for tea for example, that subject has no real interest for me. I would rather have conversation on more serious and less trivial topics, simply because speech is always such an effort for me.

Throughout the years until I left school, I received regular speech therapy, which I found hard-going, particularly when it meant that I was spending time out of class. I had to work hard to catch up and that was a perpetual struggle – thankfully in the academy my speech therapy appointments were arranged to be during a study period or physical education classes. Even into my teens, all I seemed to be required to do was to practise individual sounds – which was very frustrating and did not seem to improve my speech significantly. It was only during my mid-teens that I received speech therapy which seemed to make some real difference. By then, I was practising complete sentences and not single words. That was a step forward but even today my speech still has not reached a level where I can say that it does not hold me back in conversation.

As I have grown towards maturity, I find that my speech impairment has undoubtedly restricted me from achieving all I want from life. For example, I would love to apply for a job which mentally stimulates me but, as I have said already, any post that might do this requires effective communication skills which inevitably disqualifies me.

I find myself using very basic language when I am speaking as I do not have the opportunity to rehearse in my head what I would wish to say. When I do manage to use the kind of terminology I would prefer, I am sometimes questioned as to how I know such things. One example of that occurred at my first book launch. When Professor John Swinton was interviewing me, I was asked if he had written the script for me. Absolutely not! He would not dare to do so, because I know my own mind! I had to explain that I actually told him what I wanted to say and he wrote a set of questions accordingly. That was not the first time I had been asked if Professor Swinton had told me what to say. At our church's A.G.M. I asked a question pertaining to the balance sheets for the current and previous years. It surprised people how much detail I understood with regard to accounting. Admittedly, the specific issue concerned disability, but Professor Swinton had no idea that I was planning to ask any questions at all. Since it was a finance issue and so related to my Higher National Certificate qualification, I probably understood more of the balance-sheet calculations than did many of the others. That illustrates how so many people (even friends that know me well) do not fully appreciate how I have to modify my speech when I am talking. When I know what I am intending to say, and have worked out in advance how to say it, that preparation empowers me to be able to speak in public.

Prejudice and misunderstandings towards those with speech disabilities are not so uncommon as many might imagine. There is a Member of Parliament who has mild cerebral palsy and speech difficulties, who felt he was being ridiculed in the House of Commons. This story made the headlines in the *Times* during February 2011: it was shocking, yet thrilling, to see a paper like the *Times* take the issue so seriously. It seems to me that having a speech impairment is a topic that is seldom spoken about. Another common reaction is that people will say, 'Why don't you get speech therapy so that your speech will improve and then be like everyone else's?' What nonsense! Yes, I might receive some more speech therapy but then the issue might be – how much effort do I need to put in even to improve marginally? Simply reading about a person who is an MP with a significant speech impairment brings me real encouragement. More importantly, it makes people think about the matter and may even aid MPs to re-assess their views on the question of speech disabilities. It is good therefore that the issue has now been highlighted and existing prejudices have been challenged.

For many years, I had been bullied at school and elsewhere to varying degrees. You may ask how relevant that is to communication. It actually has much more significance than one would imagine. The more uncomfortable I feel, the more awkward my speech becomes. When this happens, I tend to become loud or else avoid talking. Being teased at school meant that I did not participate in class discussions as fully as I would have wished, had I only had enough confidence – people who know me well are often surprised how much I lack confidence due to this time in my life!

After school, I actually shortened my name to 'Kate' for about seven or eight years. I particularly wanted to do so for two reasons. The first was that people tended always to pick my name up as 'Catherine' – which really annoyed me since, no matter how hard I tried to correct them, they always persisted in saying 'Catherine'. The second reason was that every time I heard my name being spoken, it brought back memories of being bullied at school – I was almost trying to run away from that memory. My granny's name on Mum's side was 'Kate-Ann' and so 'Kate' seemed a natural choice, having always known I was called after her. It was not until I was buying my flat, and kept finding my full name being written and spoken, that the wounds began to heal. Now I really like my own name and dislike being called 'Kate' because that reminds me of how much I had almost to become another person in order to break with memories of the past. I do have one good friend, however, whom I allow to call me 'Kate' – and that is Brian Irvine, the ex-Dons football player. Brian is a close friend and when I met him I was calling myself 'Kate' and it is nice to know that, when I meet Brian at a public event and people hear him saying 'Kate', they realise he does know me very well. Apart from Brian and a few family members who call me 'Kate', I try to insist that everyone else calls me 'Kathleen' as my speech surely is not so bad that they cannot make my name out properly.

I love talking and always have. People often remark that I 'never shut up' but actually I only talk a lot if I know I am in the company of people who accept me for who I am. When I need to make 'small-talk' or polite conversation with people, I do not really know how to do it and it becomes a great effort. Making friends is very difficult unless we share something in common to start with.

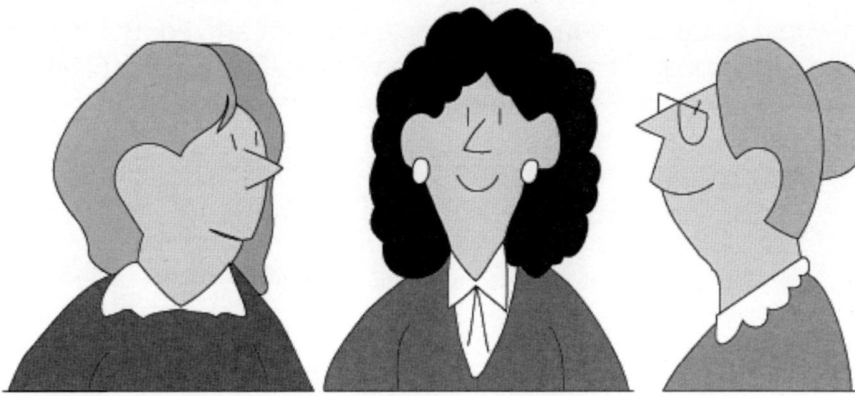

USING THE TELEPHONE

I recall being young and the question being asked whether I would ever be able to use a telephone when I grew up. Gradually, as I went through primary and into secondary school, I began to answer the phone at home, and many of the comments I would get were really interesting and encouraging. Some people even today say I am actually clearer on the phone than in face-to-face conversation – which surprises me! I believe this is because people are only hearing me speak and are not actually looking at my face being distorted while I talk.

Using a telephone was going to prove vital at some points in my life. One of the best examples occurred when I choked on a sausage while at home in my flat. I realised I was beginning to panic. Not sure how bad I was, I rang my Uncle Graham in his shop and was able to find just enough breath to let him know that I was at home. Thankfully, his shop is only five minutes from my flat and he came immediately to my assistance. The reason I hadn't phoned the ambulance was that I kept thinking the sausage I had choked on would come up even before Uncle Graham arrived. But it hadn't – the sausage didn't emerge until we were half-way to hospital! This wasn't the only time something like this happened, but I am grateful that I can indeed use the phone.

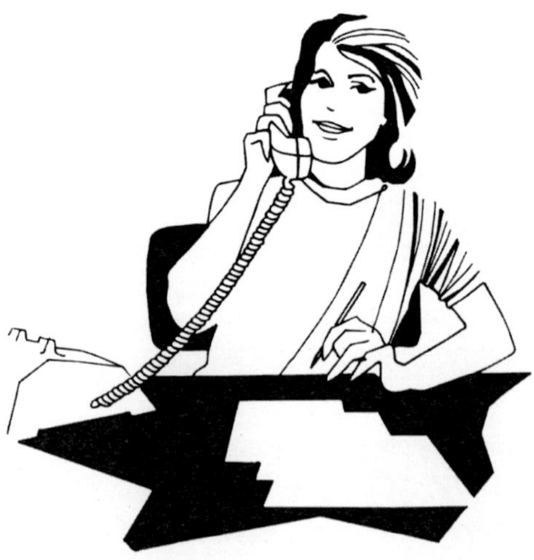

WRITING

During my early school years and up until the end of first year at secondary school, whenever I wrote anything, I had to abbreviate what I wanted to say. The sheer physical effort of putting my thoughts on to paper was enough of a struggle, without having to elaborate on the content. The entire frustration was uppermost in my mind and often upset me – as it does even today. No one else realised this until I began studying for my Open University degree and became brave enough to use certain terms that I had acquired through studying.

My written communication is severely impaired in comparison to my speech – something that is not well known. This is partly for the reasons given above but more so because I have never truly learned how. By that, I mean I can tell you the spelling rules like 'i before e except after c' but in primary school, all my efforts were focused on setting the words on to the page and by the end of first year in secondary, I had a scribe. The reason I did not use a typewriter or word-processor or lap-top, was that technology was not so advanced at that time. In any case, learning to communicate through the written word was enough for my powers of concentration without having to type at the same time.

Eight or nine years ago, when we were running the prayer group at work and writing 'Thought of the Week', I began to realise that mentally I knew what I wanted to say but I could not set it down effectively on paper. I wrote, but felt as if the wording was very 'childish' since I was trying to avoid using any technical terms. I could not share deep insights with the person I had asked to correct my grammar unless they could place the same interpretation as me on what was written. This was often frustrating. Again, as with my speech, it meant that what I would actually write was not really how I wanted to portray my message.

Now that I am studying for an Open University degree, I find I actually understand what I am studying but transcribing my meaning on to paper is the hardest part. I realise that might well be the case for many others, but for me it is especially frustrating.

Does this curtail me in employment? Yes, since when I see a job description which demands 'good verbal and written communication skills', that tends to disqualify me again.

It was once suggested that I should use a microphone and talk into a computer which would translate everything I said instead of my trying to type it. Because of my speech difficulties, it would take so long for the machine to get used to my voice that it would not be worth the effort. At the moment I keep trying to improve my grammar and spelling in any way I can.

Do I have dyslexia? Probably, but it is far more complicated with my speech impairment being as it is. I do use a program on my laptop, which reads back everything I write but it is not ideal. I am sure that in the future, there will be new software that will help to improve this. To have software that reads just like a human voice would make such a difference but I feel we have a long way to go! The software I have is acceptable on WORD or a PDF but not really adequate when reading online or sending emails, so it can be very frustrating.

Another problem I have when I am writing is that I actually omit words. I have never managed to decide whether I am thinking too far in advance or whether I don't realise that I have missed out a word. Again, this could actually be tied in with the way I speak but I am honestly not sure. What I can tell you is that, if someone (not the computer!) actually reads it aloud for me, I can usually tell where most of the mistakes are and how I can correct them. It does frustrate me, however, that the computer software is not sophisticated enough and that my disability is still holding me back. I can honestly say, when it comes to my OU exams, that I do struggle with this, but the alternative is to have a scribe. The regulations state that a scribe would require to be someone that I don't know – which would just complicate matters more. My exams are nearly four hours long, since extra time is allocated due to my disability, and on top of that, I have fifteen minutes break per hour. The sheer effort of speaking for that length of time would be virtually impossible for me (and anyone else!)

Emailing and texting

In recent years, there have been new ways of communicating: namely texting from a mobile phone and emailing. Texting is very casual and shared between friends; emailing can also be casual but it can also be formal, depending on the context of the email. I have a friend abroad to whom I used to hand-write letters regularly for a number of years. When I wrote those letters, I always tried to use my best grammar – this used to take ages! Nowadays, I simply email them – for some reason it is a lot easier – I don't panic about grammar or spelling. I suppose it is more acceptable for an email not to be perfect, which is beneficial to me, as that gives me a greater sense of independence. Previously I had to ask someone to check my grammar, before I could send the letter. Nowadays, I just send it! Texting, the other new form of communication, is widely used today. Texting is almost a completely new language and some of the abbreviations are actually very like the ones I used when I was at school, which I find amusing!

I find that people are often puzzled and sceptical when they first hear that my grammar is affected by my disability. At the moment, I receive grammar tuition and help with my writing once a week, which has made a difference, encouraging me to use more sophisticated language when I am writing, because I am shown how to correct it.

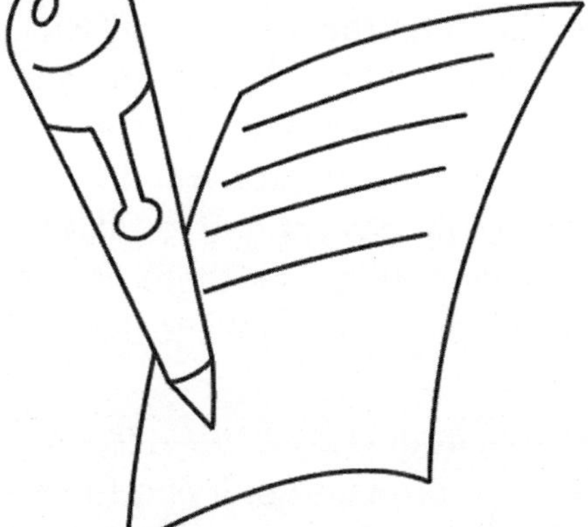

CHRISTMAS

When I am asked if I love Christmas time, I have to say 'No!' The media, of course, would have us believe that we all should thoroughly enjoy this season – yet Christmas has become little more than a commercial extravaganza, and one that seems to arrive earlier each year. When my parents ran their own shop, I recall going with them to a Christmas trade fair in March! That only serves to show that retailers have to plan several months ahead when they are ordering goods for Christmas. Some shops begin to display Christmas cards in August and so the annual commercial hype is on its way by early autumn.

Christmas itself is an extremely difficult time for me personally, with the emphasis being placed very much on making light, social conversation with family or with friends whom we may not see at any other time of the year. It seems that everything of a serious kind stops – normal working routines cease, as do regular activities like prayer meetings and study groups – which results in there being less structure to every part of my daily life. I thrive on routine and discipline, so that Christmas disrupts that sense of regularity.

As a child, I always enjoyed the build-up to Christmas but, by the time it arrived, I was either over-excited or had already had enough and just wished the festivities were all over. Of course, my parents' shop was open in the mornings on Christmas Day and New Year's Day with the rest of the time in between being 'business as usual', which helped keep the celebrations low-key while I was a teenager. When very young, however, I would become completely over-awed on Christmas Day by all the presents. I simply did not know how to appreciate them, nor could I comprehend all the toys – it was all just far too much for me! Mum always had to take them away, and then begin very gradually to re-introduce them one by one. That always seemed to work – other parents might find this solution works equally well for them.

Even now, Christmas frequently ends in tears for me and I believe that is simply due to the pressure of trying to be sociable. I suspect many others may also feel this but deal with it differently. Now that

I am older, and live independently, I am often asked whether I will be going home for Christmas. The simple answer is that I am at home in my own flat! Yet there is always a good deal of pressure to conform and to participate in the general 'season of goodwill'.

At work, there is always much excitement during the Christmas period and I would do almost anything to avoid it. I do go to the office Christmas lunch, but try hard to steer clear of anything else in the way of celebration.

For me, Christmas is a religious festival and that is what the entire celebration ought to be about – rejoicing that God became flesh as a baby. I have a friend who said she always disliked Christmas, despite being a committed Christian. I used to think that was very strange – but now I can honestly say that I wholly agree with her.

I do attend all the Christmas services at my church, but sometimes I feel I am doing so because that is what is expected of me. Give me Easter any day! I much prefer that time of celebration.

Over the past two years, my church elder has become accustomed to sending me some form of task on Christmas Eve – I notice it arriving in my e-mail inbox and immediately think of it as something to be completed over the festive period – a strange Christmas gift you may say – but very welcome to me!

The task is always quite unrelated to Christmas: but what a difference it is to be presented with a challenge which stimulates me mentally and stops me being preoccupied with the time of year.

Sometimes I work on my Open University studies, and that invariably keeps me fruitfully occupied.

Whenever I look on Facebook on the internet or meet up with friends around this time of year, they are always talking about 'this party' or 'that party'. In some respects, I would like to be invited, but for so many other reasons I am very glad that I am not.

Naturally we all enjoy opening the gifts we receive, but when I was a very small child, it was extremely difficult for my parents to buy suitable toys for me. Certain toys were quite unsuitable for me because of my lack of dexterity – they were far too awkward for me to handle. One Christmas present which has always been memorable, however, was a Tiny Tears doll which I could handle easily and with which I played for many years.

Now that I am older, presents are probably even more difficult for my family to choose for me. Jewellery is unsuitable – not because I dislike it (like most women I love jewellery) but because I am unable to put it on by myself. I have been given so many necklaces and bracelets in the past, yet sadly they just lie unused in their boxes. If I were going out somewhere with a friend or family member, I could ask them to fasten a necklace for me, but it would be vital to remember to ask them to unfasten it afterwards. Make-up is another present I used to receive from friends (but my family knew better!). At one point, I had two or three shelves of make-up, which were never touched – but fortunately those days are long past. As we grow older, we tend to stop buying make-up for one another. One present, of course, that never goes wrong for me is anything in the toiletry line, as I find the best way for me to relax in an evening, after work or study, is to have a hot bubble-bath. That helps to ease the muscular tension which I find is hard to relieve at the best of times, but a bath always seems to do the trick. A bath is more suitable for me than a shower because I am lying down and not having to stand and reach up while washing my hair. That certainly throws me off balance if I am not very careful. I do enjoy a shower though if I am away from home, knowing that if I don't reappear, someone will come along to check that I haven't slipped and fallen.

The 28th of December is my godson's birthday and that always brings me great joy. It feels so natural an event and, instead of focusing on all the Christmas hype, I can concentrate on Alasdair's birthday!

At New Year, Mum usually prepares a big New Year dinner for family and friends – undoubtedly the best way for us to handle that annual celebration.

This account serves to illustrate how severely I am affected by my disability at a time when most people are making merry. When I organise my life, I am able to do so very satisfactorily – except for

Christmas. I am so very grateful that my family and close friends know how much I struggle at this time and how hard they try to make sure that there is no undue pressure on me to become over-excited.

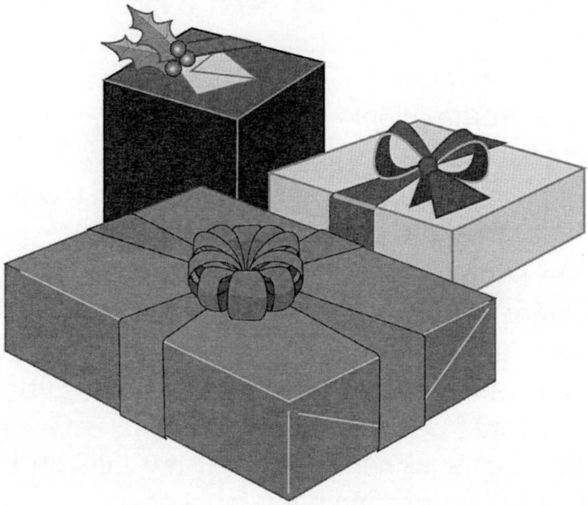

BIRTHDAYS

Age is an achievement that one should not take for granted nor is it something that is embarrassing!

In my previous book, I mentioned how I was extremely ill and very near to death just after I was born. To have been in the Special Unit fighting for my life does make me think very seriously about how precious life is. Only after I had been baptised did my fragile life seem to gain enough strength to fight for existence. Until then, there had been a question about my survival and indeed what my quality of life would be. Some people who believe in euthanasia may argue that only certain lives are worth living and they would not have rated mine as being sufficiently worthwhile to justify all the specialists' help that has been required to give me a quality of life.

It is said one should never ask a lady her age. Well, I take great delight in my age! When I reveal my age, folk are often shocked either by how old I am or how young I am. A funny story occurred when my Uncle Graham was talking to the *Evening Express* before my book launch and he said I was twenty-eight. It was amusing because he had been the master of ceremonies at my thirtieth birthday party, over five years before my first book launch!

I must say, I usually celebrate all my birthdays in some way, as I see them all as landmarks – the usual form is celebrating with the whole family as my birthday lands between that of my brother Calum Murdo and of my Uncle Graham, whose birthdays are a week apart. It is a birthday week but usually the celebrations are combined somehow – which is great fun.

All my 'big' birthdays – 18, 21 and 30 – have been celebrated with large parties, each one being completely different. My eighteenth was a disco at which we forgot to cut the birthday cake. There was not much structure to it, but I danced the whole evening – I love dancing. When I was twenty-one, we organised the same kind of party, but this time some friends, Henry and Hazel Irvine-Fortescue, put on a puppet show telling the gospel story. It helped to give the night some structure and most people enjoyed it.

For my thirtieth birthday party I had decided that this should enable all my friends and family to see different facets of my life. How I organised this was to have a selection of friends, in whom I trusted, to speak about how they knew me and in what context. This was interesting for my friends and family as I had compartmentalised my life so well that there were some who had no idea of other parts of my life until that night. I found this was definitely the easiest party so far, as there was structure as well as time for dancing. Anyone who might question the quality of life I would have just needs to be around when I am hosting one of my big birthday parties – and all will be revealed.

Birthday parties, even when I was younger, were always faced with mixed emotions – particularly if it was someone else's party. I would feel very inadequate compared to the other girls for some reason. I do remember sometimes being in a panic about having to ask for a non-paper cup at the party – stupid really, but it felt so important at the time! Obviously, at any of my own parties, a cup was already placed on the table where I was to be sitting. Birthday parties or celebrations seem to become less structured as we grow older and I find it more difficult to make polite small-talk!

Some birthday parties which I have attended as an adult have been ceilidhs. I enjoy ceilidh dancing because there is structure to each set dance, but having said that, I enjoy dancing, full stop! Sometimes at ceilidhs or other parties, people are quite surprised to see me dance – they seem to be worried in case I fall. If this happens, I just pick myself up and carry on. Being serious though, I am careful when dancing not to move too quickly. I just think to myself that they will appreciate a slower pace as some dances can go on for quite a while.

Celebrating birthdays has a significant meaning for me and I have a saying that sums it up –

A life worth living is a life worth celebrating!

RELATIONSHIPS

Relationships make up a very high proportion of all our lives, and this is one area that I struggle with because of my disability. During the teenage years most young people gradually learn how to socialise with their peers and seniors. Although as a child, I learned to respect people in authority, yet nowadays I am at times almost frightened by them.

People sometimes confuse acquaintanceship and friendship, but they are essentially different. An acquaintance is somebody we know casually to greet in the passing – without there being any emotional attachment. A friend, on the other hand, is someone you care for and who reciprocates the feeling.

I naturally have dozens, indeed hundreds, of acquaintances, as do most people. For me these are people with whom I am in touch either through church or work or social networks such as Facebook. Over the years, I have acquired another kind of acquaintance: a person who has met me only once or has heard about me through a friend or by way of an organisation. There was one lady whom I used to encounter when I was in town on a Saturday. She always spoke to me as if I had known her and her daughter from nursery days. I did not remember her at all, and consequently I always found this encounter quite embarrassing since she would compare me with her own daughter who had an entirely different form of disability. The simplest way of avoiding such occurrences was for me to stop going into town on Saturdays as I found the meetings so awkward.

It is still very hard for me to make friends. As I explained in the Communication section, making small-talk is very difficult for me. The obvious way for me to make friends is to meet with others having a shared interest, as I then know what to talk about.

If I were not studying with the Open University, I would attend our local branch of the Bible Study Fellowship which is an interdenominational study course for women. I loved being involved with this before concentrating on my OU studies.

As the emphasis was always on topics from the Bible, it was a simple matter to build up friendships based on that. Although the work involved was always demanding (about six hours of homework per week), I found it was easy to talk with people who had studied the same topic. In the course of our discussion it was simple to move on to other matters of common interest.

I find it easier to keep friendships within somewhat formal boundaries. By this I mean that there needs to be a certain element of structure to the friendship. Any friendship which is simply based on light-hearted socialising is very hard-going so far as I am concerned. To be honest, there is not a great deal one can say about the weather! Having such boundaries offers a degree of protection for myself (and others). Otherwise I find myself unintentionally sharing personal details and end up divulging information I had planned to keep to myself.

I also have boundaries of another kind which may seem unusual. I 'compartmentalise' my friends because I feel quite uncomfortable having the same friends in different facets of my life. I have certainly a small group of friends who know me in varied situations, but those are generally close friends who do understand fully that this is the only way I can handle my relationships. That may seem hard but it ensures that I am in control of my life. It may sound as if I am some kind of control freak, yet I am not. It is just my personal defence-mechanism for coping. It seems to work for me, although others sometimes find it strange.

Conflicting ironically with this method of coping with different friendships, my minister at present knows most of my mother's family and is aware of some of the family history. This is comforting in many ways, as he has often reminded me of my rich church background. Coincidentally, my church elder is acquainted with several of the specialists who helped me when I was younger. However, neither my minister nor my elder raises a topic of that nature unless I have done so first – and certainly never in front of others.

Still, church fellowship is hard, as there is so much expectation to make small-talk, which I can manage only if I am feeling on top form.

So far as family matters are concerned, I allow few friends to become closely involved, for this is an area of my life that I really treasure and like to keep very private. That probably stems from the fact that the members of my family have been so supportive and have never drawn attention to my disability. I recall someone once asking if they might pray that my parents could believe that I would be healed. This upset me greatly because the person concerned failed to understand that I was loved just as I was.

I have another good friend that I am happy to have around at any time. This is my godson Alasdair, who now plays a very important part in my life. Although still very young, he accepts me just as I am. To him I am at all times 'Auntie Kathleen' and he brings me such joy in the way he has accepted me. Whether I am playing with him, reading to him or even praying for him, he just loves me.

When I was a child, it was common for adults (and may still be) to ask, 'Who is your boyfriend?' or 'Haven't you found a boyfriend yet?' As one grows older, people tend to stop asking that, yet for some strange reason I am still asked such questions. I honestly do not think they realise how insensitive that is. I actually find it very hurtful at times, but I do realise they do not mean to be offensive.

Allowing someone access to all the secrets and intimate aspects of one's life can be more than a little daunting! It would certainly be an enormous challenge for me if I were to share such details with a partner! I simply have to trust that God may provide the right man for me – someone who is capable of understanding how I cope with relationships.

As you may now understand, relationships form a difficult area of my life – one which requires me to be disciplined and alert – even at times when you would expect me to be relaxed and completely at ease. Perhaps it seems a strange strategy; but it works for me!

EXERCISE AND RELAXATION

Anyone who knows me will be aware that I never stop. My mother once said that I never sit down. Believe me, I am never fully at rest unless I have something that requires me to be still.

As I have mentioned in my earlier book, just after I was born, the hospital did not give me much hope of survival, but I seemed to gain more strength after I was baptised. For me, life is for living – and living it to the full! This may explain my need to be either on-time or earlier for any meetings which I am attending, or whenever I am planning to meet someone. Another reason for good time-keeping is that if I am ever late in arriving, it raises alarm bells that something may have happened to me.

<u>Exercise</u>

When I was younger and receiving physiotherapy, it was always carried out in front of a mirror. There is nothing like a mirror to emphasise how different one's movements are – believe me! Even as a child at the Raeden Centre, I used to dread having physiotherapy. Yes, I do understand why physiotherapy is performed in front of a mirror – so as to help with posture – but it horrified me. When I move, I do not realise how all my movements are exaggerated compared to those of others. When I brush my hair, I brush it without a mirror, except for the final touches to ensure it is sitting correctly. I have been asked many times whether I rehearse in front of a mirror before speaking in public. I do not – the reason being that it would put me off.

I find it interesting that physiotherapy was always performed in front of a mirror, yet speech therapy and occupational therapy were not. This was something that puzzled me, but I have since been told that sometimes speech therapy is practised in front of a mirror. I would have found the distortion in my face quite off-putting if I had had to use a mirror.

My favourite activities are walking, horse-riding and swimming. I do enjoy going for walks as long as I am not under any duress, as this can make me quite stiff and liable to fall with the risk of doing some physical damage to myself. On the other hand, I would always rather walk than drive if I am stressed, as I am less expensive to fix than any car!

Both horse-riding and swimming are activities which need to come either at the end of the day or at the start, due to the effort of undressing and then dressing again. Swimming in particular exhausts me, due to the effort I have to put in, particularly if the swimming pool is cold.

Swimming, however, is something I have always enjoyed. I even recall being in the small swimming pool at Raeden Nursery and going through some of my physiotherapy there. Being in water always relaxes my muscles. Interestingly, my difficulties with saliva are never evident after that.

My regular sporting activity is to go horse-riding – which is very expensive. In fact, it costs nearly one pound per minute, but then we do know that I have expensive tastes – at least in shoes and hobbies! When I tell people that I go horse-riding weekly, I would say that nine out of ten are surprised. I wonder why – I suspect people can't imagine I would do anything so dangerous as that, but I would try anything at least once – life is for living! Nothing can compare with the freedom I enjoy when I am trotting or cantering. The only thing which comes near to it, is when, as a child, I used to go sledging down a steep hill in Findon which would be all covered with snow in the winter. That was thrilling and gave me an immense sense of freedom.

Relaxation

Do I ever relax? The question perhaps should be, "Do I know what the word 'relax' means?" Probably not. I am always on the go. There are only two places where I relax: in the bath and in my bed. I have written about bathing in another chapter so I won't repeat myself. Being unable to relax is partly due to my cerebral palsy but another reason may be that I have inherited this from my mother's side of the family, who were crofters on the island of Lewis and Harris, where there was always much work to be done from sheer necessity.

If I want to unwind or am ill and unable to be as active as I normally like to be, I enjoy doing jigsaw puzzles – which is quite amazing, considering my lack of dexterity. I do have to be careful, however, when I begin to tackle a new one, since it can end up consuming all my spare time – and becoming very addictive. This is a hobby that I like to share with my friends, Emma and Mike, and I know that every Christmas, when I go and see them, there will always be one lying out. Usually we end up completing it while I am there!

At times, when I am needing a break from studying or writing, I may play a card game on my laptop. This involves playing solitaire with four different packs of cards.

The sheer diversity and complexity of my disability may be quite apparent in quite diverse and unexpected ways, contrary to what many might imagine.

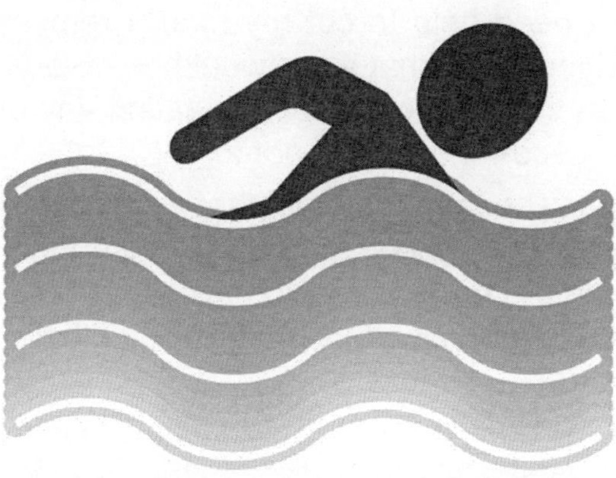

CAFÉS AND RESTAURANTS

I love to eat out, particularly if it is somewhere with a pleasant ambience. A supermarket café is not classed as 'eating out' in my opinion; it is simply having a bite to eat for convenience. I enjoy my food, especially if someone else has cooked it.

My family always liked going out somewhere for a meal. I recall when I was a teenager, or even younger, being in restaurants or cafés and realising that I appeared to be the only person there who was physically disabled. Thankfully, this is no longer the case today.

When I was a teenager, after my parents' shop had closed for the night, we sometimes went up to Portlethen Golf Club along with my uncle Graham. In those days, the kitchen closed at nine. Some might say that they kept it open just for us as our shop only closed at half past eight in the evening. Eating out was an important part of our lives then.

I have always found it a hassle when dining in a restaurant without my family, as I need help to cut my food. I remember being in a restaurant and forgetting that there would be no one to help cut my meal for me, so that I ended up barely eating any of it. This taught me a valuable lesson which I will not forget.

Some time ago, I began to notice that when one ordered a pizza in an Italian restaurant, the waiters were more than willing to cut it into manageable pieces. Some automatically offer this service when they realise that I have poor hand control and others are very willing to oblige if asked.

An amusing incident occurred this summer when I went out for lunch with my brother Calum Murdo to an Italian restaurant. I ordered a pizza and of course it had already been cut into segments when served at our table. When I ordered a Coca-Cola, I also asked for a straw. My brother had not thought about a straw and had simply asked for an empty glass as he presumed that he would need to pour half of my Coke into the empty glass.

Obviously, he did not need to do so and, with the pizza having already been cut, he looked rather puzzled, as if to say: “What can I do? It has all been done.” Calum Murdo’s own life has been affected in so many ways due to my cerebral palsy but, like my own, it would be hard to imagine it any other way. Other restaurants are now offering this type of service.

When I was at Holyrood, I wonder what would have happened if I had asked for my meal to be cut up before it was brought to the table. I knew that either Professor Swinton or Lewis Macdonald MSP would be willing to assist me and that therefore I did not need to ask. Throughout the day at Holyrood, there were various instances like this – which I believe may have prompted Professor Swinton to challenge me to write this book.

As time goes on, I hope to find more restaurants being prepared to help their customers by offering to portion the food before it arrives at the table. This is such a great help and I feel so much more comfortable knowing that it will come prepared for me without my having to rely on someone else.

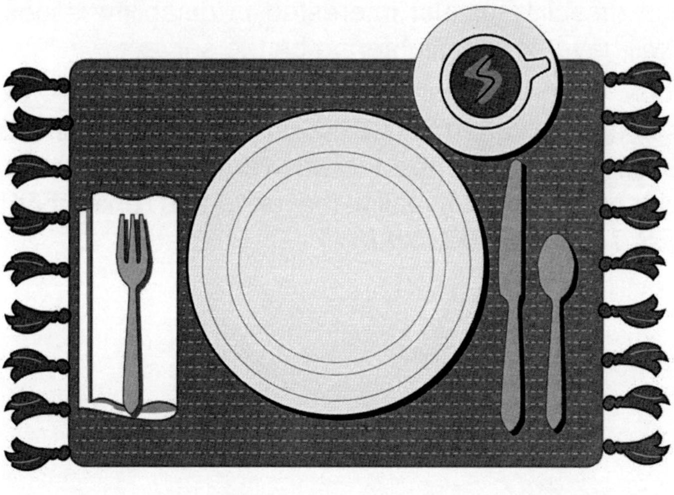

EPILOGUE: WHAT NOW?

Drawing my book to a conclusion should not suggest that all the difficulties have disappeared or that there is nothing more to say. If the contents of this small book have given some insight into disability, my hope is that it may encourage people to change their perceptions and perhaps rethink their ideas concerning disability.

For myself, I hope over the next two years to complete my degree with the Open University. That certainly will be an achievement! However, once qualified, I would hope to be able to help others to understand that the attitude 'Yes I can and I will' is an extremely important principle when people with disabilities are faced with obstacles every day.

If there are no work opportunities immediately arising from this, I suspect I will begin studying for a Psychology degree since, whenever I have studied psychology in my BA Hons in Business Studies, I have found this subject particularly interesting. This illustrates how much I continually try to stretch my brain.

By reading these chapters, whether you are someone with a recognised disability or just interested in disability issues, I hope that you will have been enlightened on the subject.

This book may demonstrate that when people are examining disability issues, it is often the most ordinary tasks which prove to be the most difficult. Even when the answers aren't always apparent, people with or without a disability may stop and remember the book called ***YES, I CAN, AND I WILL.***